LOOK BETTER.
FEEL BETTER.
LIVE BETTER.

What God Wants You to Know About Food

by

D.A. Justice

Scripture taken from the HOLY BIBLE, NEW INTERNATIONAL VERSION®. NIV®. Copyright © 1973, 1978, 1984 by International Bible Society. Used by permission of Zondervan. All rights reserved worldwide.

The information provided in this book is designed to provide helpful information on the subjects discussed. This book is not meant to be used, nor should it be used, to diagnose or treat any medical condition. This book is designed to provide information and motivation to the customer. For diagnosis or treatment of any medical problem, consult your own physician. The author is not responsible for any specific health or allergy needs that may require medical supervision and is not liable for any damages or negative consequences from any treatment, action, application or preparation, to any person reading or following the information in this book. No warranties or guarantees are expressed or implied by the author's choice to include any of the content in this book. The author shall not be liable for any physical, psychological, emotional, financial, or commercial damages, including, but not limited to, special, incidental, consequential or other damages. References are provided for informational purposes only and do not constitute endorsement of any other sources. You are responsible for your own choices, actions, and results.

Look Better. Feel Better. Live Better.
What God Wants You to Know About Food
ISBN: 978-0-9994436-0-6
Copyright © 2018 by D.A. Justice

Published by Word and Spirit Publishing
P.O. Box 701403
Tulsa, Oklahoma 74170
wordandspiritpublishing.com

Cover copyright © 2017 by D.A. Justice Ministries.
Cover design by Joshua I. Justice.

Printed in the United States of America. All rights reserved under International Copyright Law. Content and/or cover may not be reproduced in whole or in part in any form without the expressed written consent of the Publisher.

To Joshua and Joseph—
you are the arrows in my quiver.

Mom, your never-yielding love and support
were my sail in many a storm. Thanks, Ma.

To my pastor, Dr. W.C. Turner,
and to my Mt. Level Missionary Baptist
Church family,
thank you for opening the door.

To my Lillington Star Church family,
I am the luckiest pastor
in the world.

CONTENTS

Foreword ix

Introduction xi

Balanced Blessings 1

    A Good Foundation 3
    It Works 6
    Back to the Future 12
    Closing Prayer 20

Taste and See 23

    A Heavenly Health Plan 27
    On-the-Way Blessings 37
    Closing Prayer 38

God's Food Ain't Cheap 41

    Looking for a Miracle 43
    In Jesus' Hands 47
    Closing Prayer 56

Fellowship of a Miracle 59

    A Renewed Image 60
    Change of Attitude 62
    Closing Prayer 70

"Almost, Not Yet" 73

    Strength While You Wait 75
    Blessed Food 83
    Closing Prayer 85

The Children's Crumbs 89

    Don't Forget the Oil 90
    She Called Him "Lord" 96
    Closing Prayer 102

Epilogue: Slay It 105

Scripture Meditations 107

Additional Resources 109

TABLES

Leafy Greens and Benefits...13

Fruit and Benefits 16

Nuts and Benefits 19

Herbs and Benefits 34

Whole Grain and Benefits..52

Whole Grain and Benefits..99

Fish and Benefits..55

Grass-Fed Meats and Benefits..68

(Anti-Aging) Fruit and Benefits..82

Oil and Benefits 95

FOREWORD
by
W.C. Turner, Ph.D.
Duke University

Dr. Derrick Justice has made a splendid offering in this book that intersects spiritual and physical health around the subject of eating well. He has revisited the truths of how our good God has furnished the creation with wonderful offerings of sustenance and healing, showing how good choices made in food bless us in countless ways. The benefits, which are both spiritual and physical, come to rest when we embrace the unity of our obedience and glorify God in our bodies. We need this wholeness which has been provided to obey God in our callings more fully and to set an example and lead the way for others seeking patterns that lead to victory. It is a wonderful and refreshing read. It preaches and teaches us as we glide through its pages. It sets at our fingertips the very blessings that we need and that we need to pass along to others. Many stand to benefit from this choice offering.

INTRODUCTION

We live totally in a culture of bad food. From humongous hamburgers to fried pickles, we are inundated with bad food choices. Unhealthy eating is made so cheap and easy today that there's no wonder why so many of us give in to temptation and simply just go with the flow: overeat, gain weight, that's just the way it is. The quality and quantity of bad food is so prevalent in our society that not only has it wreaked havoc on our physiology, but it has drastically diminished our psychology. We have accepted as normal bloated bellies, wide butts, and the resulting chronic illnesses associated with both, and the way we eat harbors most of the blame.

Our faith, however, is still the most powerful and beautiful expression of the godly life we have. God has given us a measure of faith, and He intends for it to be bodacious. So, why limit it? Sadly, too many of us limit our faith in the one key area of life that is crucial to how we look, feel, and live: our food. This book reveals how to apply faith strategically to the food we eat in order to get the life we want.

Other than the courtesy grace spoken over the typical meal, most of us have totally relegated our food and how we generally think about diet and nutrition to the realm of secular specialists and experts. Fortunately, God has so much to say about the food we eat and how we should think about our dietary habits, and it's all just waiting to be unlocked and engaged. This book presents the key to better.

In this revelatory book, faith and food collide, creating an explosive experience that will transform the way people look at food and think about what they eat. The faithful will walk away from this experience empowered to get their bodies back, their health back, and their lives back.

First and foremost, real food comes from heaven, and the goodness found in food is there because God put it there for His people. Well the latest research shows that good and whole food is packed with all kinds of disease-fighting capabilities. Unfortunately, too many of us are unaware of the blessings of food and what is at our disposal in the food choices we make. Instead, we blindly eat unhealthily, resulting in many of the chronic illnesses that plague so many people of the world.

From a unique corrective lens, this book shows the reader how God intends for food to be employed to initiate total wellness into a person's life. With opened eyes and awakened faith, the reader will see food from a new perspective that will impact eating habits and will deliver and set free from the debilitating and overpowering cravings associated with poor food choices.

People searching for answers to health and wellness through food will walk away from this enjoyable, thoroughly-researched, often-humorous and unique reading experience equipped with knowledge about which foods deliver amazing results and how to incorporate them faithfully into their diets. The benefits associated with the foods as outlined in this book have been documented and widely accepted by health experts and nutritionists alike from all over the world.

The reader of this book, who applies in faith the God-given wisdom that lies herein, is about to embark on the journey of looking better, feeling better, and living better to the glory of God.

May God richly bless you.

LOOK BETTER.
FEEL BETTER.
LIVE BETTER.

What God Wants You
to Know About Food

1

BALANCED BLESSINGS

"Eat well, love unapologetically, pray with true intention, and take care of yourself."

—Brea Herrera

One day—as pastors typically do—a colleague and I were lamenting over all the bad news on television: another police officer had killed an innocent motorist over an altercation that started because of a routine traffic stop; a prisoner out on parole brutally murdered an innocent police officer who was a single parent; politicians are more and more interested in empty rhetoric and castigating blame than they are in finding solutions. Today it seems as if the negative news cycles never end. I often wonder, "Lord, where is society headed?"

After what seemed like total exasperation on our parts, my friend stated, "God! Nobody cares. What are we going to do?" There was an ominous silence to the gravity of his question.

Upon a period of private reflection—which seemed like an eternity—we both said we are going to have to care for ourselves.

The prophet Hosea says, "My people are destroyed for a lack of knowledge" (Hosea 4:6), meaning the people in his time were being destroyed because the priests were not teaching them God's word. Typically, when we look at the ills of society and we see people being destroyed for one reason or the other, we talk about what's destroying them: community frustrations, domestic policies, drugs and violence, for example. Put another way, we focus on events. We discuss and lament over the news. However, God says that's not the issue: The issue is that the people are being destroyed because they don't have His knowledge.

For God, when the people know better, the people will do better. God wants His people to be informed so that they will thrive and will not be destroyed. The ability to do better (personally and socially) starts with knowing what God says.

The apostle John says in the epistle entitled after him, "I wish above all things that thou mayest prosper and be in health, even as thy soul prospers" (3John 2). After careful reflection, something became particularly clear: Our physical health is connected to our spiritual health. God intends for us to have spiritual health and physical health simultaneously.

It does us no good to be blessed spiritually but totally wrecked physically. Think about it, to be blessed with a nice home and a beautiful car undercuts the purpose of the blessing if you're at home and all you can do is lay in bed because you don't feel good, or when you drive the beautiful car, the only place you go is back and forth to the doctor's office. That is not what God intended for a blessed life.

Too many of God's people are prospering spiritually but NOT physically. And the truly sad part about the current state of affairs is that too many saints have accepted lopsided blessings as normal. To be blessed spiritually but debilitated physically is lopsided. Our God is greater than that: He can bless you spiritually as well as physically. Jesus says that "whatever you ask for in prayer, believe that you have received it, and it will be yours" (Mark 11:24). That's right, "whatever"! Start today asking God for balanced blessings in your life. Ask Him to heal you physically as well as spiritually.

> TO BE BLESSED SPIRITUALLY BUT DEBILITATED PHYSICALLY IS LOPSIDED. OUR GOD IS GREATER THAN THAT: HE CAN BLESS YOU PHYSICALLY AS WELL AS SPIRITUALLY.

A GOOD FOUNDATION

So, what does the Bible really say about our health? Well the foundation to how God addresses our health is found in Genesis 1:26–29 (NIV):

> Then God said, "Let us make man in our image, in our likeness, and let them rule over the fish of the sea and the birds of the air, over the livestock, over all the earth, and over all the creatures that move along the ground.
>
> So God created man in his own image, in the image of God he created him; male and female he created them.
>
> God blessed them and said to them, "Be fruitful and increase in number; fill the earth and subdue it. Rule over the fish of the sea and the birds of the air and over every living creature that moves on the ground.

> Then God said, "I give you every seed-bearing plant on the face of the whole earth and every tree that has fruit with seed in it. They will be yours for food."

To start, notice that God gave man rule over the fish, the birds, the livestock, the earth, and every creature that moves along the ground.

Next, it should be humbly pointed out that God blessed man and gave him purpose: to be fruitful, fill the earth, and subdue it.

Finally, after giving man rule and letting him know what his purpose is, God then gave man a health plan: eat every seed-bearing plant on the face of the whole earth and every tree that has fruit with seed in it.

To the man made in His image, to the one purposed to be fruitful and to rule and subdue the earth, God gave him a health care plan involving nothing but fruits and nuts and vegetables. Then God said that this is "very good" (Genesis 1:31).

It doesn't take a whole lot of scholarly insight to see that as long as man was in faithful communion with God and as long as he ate the way God said to eat, then it was all good—no disease, no complications, no illnesses. Today it is widely acknowledged that if people were to start cooking and eating more vegetables and consuming more fruits and nuts, then we'd all be in better health and experience more overall wellness. However, an "incessant intake of highly processed junk food can damage and eventually cut [one's] life short."[1]

---

[1] Friedlander, Steven, Editor-in-Chief. "You Are What You Eat: Part 1." *100 Ways to Live to 100: Expert Advice for a Longer Life*. July 2017, p. 72.

When Adam and Eve fell from grace, they did so by disobeying God's command not to eat of the tree of the knowledge of good and evil (Genesis 2:17). Reflecting upon the story of creation, or even when it's typically taught or preached, it's always done so from the standpoint that the first family disobeyed God's order, which is absolutely correct, but God is giving us new revelation today that is just as practical as it is spiritual in that Adam and Eve also disobeyed His order as it relates to their diet: They ate something God told them not to eat.

Before reading any further, ask yourself, "Am I eating something God doesn't want me to eat?" If you are, it's robbing you of your health, and it's disrupting God's plans for your life and for your longevity. As far as we know, Adam and Eve were never meant to die (Genesis 2:17).

Adam and Eve ate what God didn't want them to eat. There are some foods in our lives that God says are perfectly okay to eat, but there are other foods that God explicitly tells us not to eat. If we want balanced blessings, i.e., spiritual and physical, we will be just as faithful in our eating as we are in our stewardship. Faithful eating helps to "prevent many kinds of chronic disease, improve physical fitness and overall wellness, and even increase our brain capacity."[2] The fact the first humans could name every living creature and be trusted to govern the earth responsibly reflected a perfection of humanity directly connected to their

> WHEN YOUR FOOD LINES UP WITH YOUR FAITH, THE POSSIBILITIES FOR YOUR LIFE ARE UNLIMITED.

---

[2] Grace, Tabitha. "Deficient Nutrition." *The Power of Superfoods*. October 2017, p. 15.

faith and their food. When your food lines up with your faith, the possibilities for your life are unlimited.

In the events that led to the fall of humanity, Eve saw that the forbidden fruit was "good for food and pleasing to the eye, and also desirable [. . .]" and the moment she and Adam ate it, they started dying. Have you ever noticed that the foods that are the worst for you are the ones that look the most desirable—sugary, oily, and salty? The colors are beautiful, and the smell of them will drive you crazy. We can't get enough of them. The US Department of Agriculture recently published a report that says on average every American consumes approximately 75 lb of sugar per year, and sugar is almost as addictive as a drug. The devil knows how to set us up to go against God's best plans for our lives.

In the same way spiritual health involves being faithful, so it is that physical health involves being equally faithful. Eat more faithfully, and God will do wonders in your life.

IT WORKS

After carefully examining the foundation of God's dietary plan for His people then as well as now, another well-known passage that establishes God's use of food in direct correlation to our health is Daniel 1:8-17 (NIV):

> But Daniel resolved not to defile himself with the royal food and wine, and he asked the chief official for permission not to defile himself this way. Now God had caused the official to show favor and sympathy to Daniel, but the official told Daniel, "I am afraid of my

lord the king, who has assigned your food and drink. Why should he see you looking worse than the other young men your age? The king would then have my head because of you.

Daniel then said to the guard whom the chief official had appointed over Daniel, Hananiah, Mishael and Azariah, "Please test your servants for ten days: Give us nothing but vegetables to eat and water to drink. Then compare our appearance with that of the young men who eat the royal food, and treat your servants accordance with what you see. So he agreed to this and tested them for ten days.

At the end of the ten days they looked healthier and better nourished than any of the young men who ate the royal food. So the guard took away their choice food and the wine they were to drink and gave them vegetables instead.

To these four young men God gave knowledge and understanding of all kinds of literature and learning. And Daniel could understand visions and dreams of all kinds.

Typically, as this text relates to food, today's church sees it in terms of what's called the "Daniel Fast." But note that Daniel is not fasting; all he's doing is choosing to eat the way God says to eat: vegetables, fruits, and nuts. Eating God's way is not a fad diet or a cute church program. Although it may be difficult to do in a culture engrossed in starchy, sugary, high-caloric foods, the Lord's way of eating is a real-life way to enjoy good and divinely beneficial foods that transform your life in amazing ways to improve overall wellness.

Daniel told the chief official, "Give us nothing but vegetables to eat and water to drink. Then compare our appearance with that of the young men who eat the royal food" (vv. 12–13). At the end of the ten days, the Bible says Daniel and his friends "looked healthier and better nourished than any of the other young men who ate the royal food" (v. 15). In fact, nutrition experts agree with scripture. "Eating more plants has major benefits for your body, slashing your risk for everything from cancer and heart disease to dementia and obesity."[3]

Eating God's way will make you healthier and you'll also look better. Daniel was not fasting; he was simply eating the way God said to eat. Daniel ate according to his faith. Food experts today refer to God's way of eating as eating "superfoods," but regardless of what you call it, most nutritionists would agree that eating more faithfully will have you feeling better and looking better in no time at all, and that's truly super.

---

[3] Gold, Sunny Sea. "Your Mission: Eat More Plants." *Dr. Oz The Good Life*. June 2017, p. 82.

*Why spend money on what does not satisfy?
Listen, listen to me, and eat what is good,
and your soul will delight in the richest of fare.*
—Isaiah 55:2

For the faithful, it should be noted that eating meat did not come into the picture until after the flood (Genesis 9:3). Rather, God originally intended for His people to live primarily on vegetables, fruits, and nuts. Eating God's way is not only wise, but it is actually practical in that research clearly shows our "ancestors lived for the most part on plants—and our bodies are designed to be fueled that way"[4] and not with a diet rich in meats. If you love fast food consider that "when you have a high intake of red and processed meats, your risk of cardiovascular diseases and cancers increase,"[5] argue nutrition experts. God's plan will make His people healthier and they'll look better than the people of the world. But not only that, God's people will be smarter: Daniel also had knowledge and understanding as a result of his choosing to eat according to his faith (Daniel 1:17). Today scientists have found that diets comprised largely of plants are extremely effective in preventing "cognitive decline and Alzheimer's disease."[6]

God is a rewarder of faith, even when it comes to faithful eating. Not only will God's people look better, be healthier, and be smarter, they will live longer. Before man started eating meat, that is, so much meat, the Bible says,

A) Adam lived 930 years
B) Seth lived 912 years
C) Enosh lived 905 years

---

[4] Gold, Sunny Sea. "Your Mission: Eat More Plants." *Dr. Oz The Good Life*. June 2017, p. 80.

[5] Friedlander, Steven, Editor-in-Chief. "The Power of Protein: Stay Strong with Smarter Protein Solutions." *100 Ways to Live to 100: Expert Advice for a Longer Life*. July 2017, p. 74.

[6] Gold, Sunny Sea. "Your Mission: Eat More Plants." p. 82.

D) Kenan lived 910 years
E) Mahalalel live 895 years
F) Jared lived 962 years
G) Enoch lived 365 years and didn't even die; God just decided to take him away
H) Methuselah lived 969 years

These wonderful representatives of people who trusted in the Lord's way lived for many, many years (Genesis 5), and the Bible never says they had diabetes, high blood pressure, or any of the other chronic illnesses that are killing us today. Eating more in line with the way God designed promotes healing; for instance, "[o]ver and over, research suggests that the optimal lifestyle for preventing disease is a diet big on plants and naturally low in animal protein."[7] If you desire to be the healthy and whole person you know you can and should be, trust in God's way of eating. It works.

Disclaimer: *Do not stop taking any medications you are currently taking under doctor's orders, but consider adding more vegetables, fruits, and nuts to your diet.*

Move toward God's health care plan, and you will be amazed at the difference it will make.

As one called to preach and teach the gospel, I am always treated with a lot of love and consideration by so many wonderful and well-meaning people. Once, while preaching out of town, a dear sister brought me a meal after a powerful service so that I wouldn't have to go out to eat later that evening. When

---

[7] Gold, Sunny Sea. "Your Mission: Eat More Plants." *Dr. Oz The Good Life.* June 2017, p. 82.

she gave me the food, she had a smile on her face a mile wide and that showed all thirty of her teeth. The dear lady brought me a white styrofoam portion box full of food, and when I took hold of it, it was so heavy it almost ripped my arm off. I had to lift it with both hands, and she was still smiling. When I finally got to my hotel room and looked inside, the meat portion of the box had fried chicken, ribs, a hot dog, and three chunks of beef with sautéed onions and gravy—and in the vegetable portion was a teaspoon of vegetables. I said to myself, "Lord Jesus, I'll perish for lack of knowledge if I eat all this meat."

BACK TO THE FUTURE

As a final word on the benefits of God's health plan, the Lord closes the Bible with a remarkable passage regarding food. In heaven there's a fruit tree, the leaves of which will be for the nourishment of God's people (Revelation 22:1–2). The Holy Spirit today reveals to God's people that when they who are called by His name get to heaven, God is going to return us to His health care plan of fruits and vegetables. The Lord won't heal us with stuffed pork chops, He won't cure us with Quanisha's "Locked-and-Loaded" macaroni and cheese, He won't soothe our aches and pains with gravy from Gilead, and He won't deliver us with Reggie's World-Famous Ribs. God will heal "the nations" with vegetables, nuts, and fruits. The leaves of the tree, i.e., the vegetables, are for the healing of His people.

We have to take care of ourselves, and the way God intends for us to do it is with His dietary health plan. So, begin to eat more vegetables, fruits, and nuts, and you will start to look better and feel better the way God always intended for you to look and feel.

Here are just a few of the leafy green vegetables available as well as how they will benefit you.

Leafy Green Vegetables	Benefits	Preparation
Kale	• Promotes healthy hair, skin, nails • Keeps eyes strong • Lowers cholesterol • Fights Type 2 diabetes • Fights cancer and promotes healthy bones	• Sauté • Steam • Raw • Bake
Cabbage	• Helps mental function and concentration • Promotes healthy hair, skin, nails • Lowers blood pressure • Fights cancer • Regulates blood sugar	• Steam • Raw • Sauté
Mustard Greens	• Detoxifies the blood • Prevents cancer • Reduces heart disease and arthritis • Ensures radiant skin • Strengthens bones • Relieves Asthma	• Steam

Leafy Green Vegetables	Benefits	Preparation
Collards	• Helps lower blood sugar levels • Grows and moisturizes hair • Regulates mood, sleep, and appetite • Lowers cholesterol • Removes carcinogens from the body • Improves digestion	• Steam • Sauté
Swiss Chard	• Prevents and treats diabetes • Fights cancer • Reduces inflammation • Supports bone health	• Salad • Sauté
Arugula	• Protects eyes • Fights osteoporosis • Beautifies skin • Boosts immune system • Promotes pre-natal health • Effects weight loss	• Salad

Leafy Green Vegetables	Benefits	Preparation
Romaine	• Defends against osteoporosis • Lowers the risk of cancer • Lowers blood pressure • Lowers cholesterol • Prevents the risk of birth defects	• Salad
Turnip Greens	• Fights cancer • Leads to good eye health • Helps with fatigue • Promotes strong bones and teeth	• Steam
Spinach	• Produces a radiant complexion • Effects good eyesight • Stops dementia • Increases muscle strength • Promotes a healthy heart • Lowers cholesterol • High in fiber • Fights cancer	• Steam • Sauté • Smoothie • Wraps

Fruits are a healthy part of any diet, and God certainly does not leave them out of His health plan. In addition to tasting good, fruits offer a myriad of healing benefits. Here are a few fruits and their spectacular benefits to consider.

Fruit	Benefits	Preparation
Apples	• Lowers risk of asthma • Lowers risk of lung cancer • Regulates blood sugar	• Fruit Smoothies • Fruit Salads • Natural
Pineapples	• Prevents Asthma • Lowers blood pressure • Combats cancer • Improves blood sugar	• Fruit Smoothies • Fruit Salads • Natural
Raspberries	• Enhances male fertility • Treats Type 2 diabetes • Makes skin look younger • Effects eye health	• Fruit Smoothies • Fruit Salads • Natural

Fruit	Benefits	Preparation
Kiwis	- Repairs body tissue - Reduces effect of aging and beautifies skin - Prevents eye disease - Lowers risk of stroke - Fights cardiovascular disease - Fights cancer	- Fruit Smoothies - Fruit Salads - Natural
Cantaloupe	- Promotes a healthy immune system - Promotes eye health - Good source of Vitamin C - Stops food cravings - Fights fatigue	- Fruit Smoothies - Fruit Salads - Natural
Blueberries	- Fights the aging process - Stimulates hair growth - Lowers cholesterol - Reduces pain - Improves cardiovascular health - Lowers risk of cancer	- Fruit Smoothies - Fruit Salads - Natural

Fruit	Benefits	Preparation
Cherries	• Regulates sleep cycle • Decreases belly fat • Boosts energy • Fights dementia • Fights Type 2 diabetes • Fights the aging process • Reduces risk of Stroke • Reduces muscle pain	• Fruit Smoothies • Fruit Salads • Natural
Peaches	• Maintains healthy skin • Fights cancer cells • Promotes eye health • Helps pregnant women • Fights stress and anxiety • Helps burn stored fat • Lowers cholesterol	• Fruit Smoothies • Fruit Salads • Natural
Plums	• Fights high blood pressure • Fights cancer • Reduces risk of Type 2 diabetes • Fights dementia • Relieves stress	• Fruit Smoothies • Fruit Salads • Natural

The health benefits of nuts have been researched and studied for years. Here are a few of the healthiest nuts and the benefits of each.

Nuts	Benefits	Preparation
Walnuts	• Reduces the risk of cancer • Fights the aging process • Improves male fertility • Supports brain health • Fights Type 2 diabetes • Stimulates hair growth • Beautifies skin • Prevents heart disease	• Lightly salted and roasted • Natural
Brazil Nuts	• Boosts testosterone • Promotes radiant skin • Helps the thyroid gland • Promotes healthy immune system	• Lightly salted and roasted • Natural
Pecans	• Boosts energy • Lowers blood pressure • Lowers cholesterol • Treats osteoporosis • Slows aging process	• Lightly salted and roasted • Natural

Nuts	Benefits	Preparation
Almonds	• Controls blood sugar • Builds up cells • Lowers blood sugar • Lowers cholesterol • Reduces hunger	• Lightly salted and roasted • Natural
Cashews	• Promotes heart health • Prevents cancer • Prevents gallstones • Enriches hair color • Relaxes nerves	• Lightly salted and roasted • Natural
Pistachios	• Lowers cholesterol • Promotes skin health • Controls Type 2 diabetes • Fights aging process	• Lightly salted and roasted • Natural

CLOSING PRAYER

Most glorious Lord, give me the grace to eat more faithfully, to prosper and to be in good health. Allow me to possess the strength to stop eating the foods that do not please You, as You extend to me the desire to eat in a manner that lines up to Your will. I stand on Your word, that as I surrender to your plan for my life, my life will reflect the wellness that comes with being more faithful.

Amen.

Insights for Looking Better: _____

_____
_____
_____
_____
_____
_____
_____
_____
_____
_____
_____
_____
_____
_____
_____

Insights for Feeling Better: _____

_____
_____
_____
_____
_____
_____

LOOK BETTER. FEEL BETTER. LIVE BETTER.

Insights for Living Better:

2

TASTE AND SEE

*"If you are always trying to be normal,
you will never know how amazing you can be."*

—Maya Angelou

When we focus on food and its use in healing, we're asking, discussing, and plumbing the depths to which we want to know what God thinks of food. Ultimately, we want to identify how God wants us to look at the food we eat.

As much as food is a basic necessity of life, it is also one of life's central metaphors. One of the great promises of the Bible comes from King Solomon: "The Lord does not let the righteous go hungry" (Proverbs 10:3). How comforting it is to know that when you put your life in God's hands and live the way He says to live, He promises to always take care of your sustenance. Later Solomon says that the "lips of the righteous nourish many," indicating that it is just as important to have spiritual food as it is to have natural food for maintaining life.

Even when Jesus taught the disciples to pray, the first order of business after praising and paying homage to God the Father was to ask the Lord for food: "Give us today our daily bread" (Matthew 6:11). Before praying for forgiveness and the grace to forgive, and even before asking to be spared from temptation and delivered from evil, Jesus says to pray for food.

The righteous eats to their hearts' content,

but the stomach of the wicked goes hungry.

—Proverbs 13:25

Food is central to life. Without food, all other manifestations and experiences of life are meaningless. So much so, the need for food is a driving force. When you're hungry, you can't think about anything else. Children who are hungry in school can't learn, and people who are hungry in church can't even focus on worshipping God. Once in the middle of a beautiful homecoming service, with guests from all over the country present, the guest preacher was in the middle of his message, and around that time the food from the fellowship hall started coming up through the vents. The whole sanctuary smelled like Swedish meatballs, fried chicken, cabbage, and peach cobbler. The next thing I knew was that preacher said, "Folks, I been preaching to Black folk all my life, and I know when y'all start smelling food you're ready to go." Two minutes later he closed the message, blessed the food, and we all headed downstairs to eat. Food is a driving force even to the point of challenging a person's faith.

*So do not worry, saying,
    "What shall we eat?"*

*or "What shall we drink?" or
    "What shall we wear?"*

For the pagans run after all these things,

*and your heavenly Father knows that
    you need them.*

*But seek first his kingdom and his
    righteousness,*

*and all these things will be given
    to you as well.*

—Matthew 6:31–33

When people get hungry enough, they will disregard their faith for the sake of getting something to eat. But when people separate their faith from their food, they miss the beauty and majesty of God.

> WE TYPICALLY SEE FOOD AS SOMETHING WE DESIRE AND CRAVE; GOD SEES FOOD AS SOMETHING MEANT TO HEAL. FOOD FITS INTO THE PURPOSE OF GOD.

We typically see food as something we desire and crave; God sees food as something meant to heal. Food fits into the purpose of God. When we look at food the way God looks at food, we are ushered into blessings and healing.

A HEAVENLY HEALTH PLAN

To understand the breadth and beauty of the Bible, it is helpful to realize God's word is couched in context. The Bible is written as the story of salvation, pointing to Jesus Christ and faithful obedience to him.

> In the desert the whole community grumbled against Moses and Aaron. The Israelites said to them, "If only we had died by the Lord's hands in Egypt! There we sat around pots of meat and ate all the food we wanted, but you have brought us out into this desert to starve this entire assembly to death."
>
> Then the Lord said to Moses, "I will rain down bread from heaven for you. The people are to go out each day and gather enough for that day. In this way I will test the and see whether they will follow my instructions . . . The people of Israel called the bread

manna. It was white like coriander seed and tasted like wafers made with honey."

Exodus 16:2–4, 31 (NIV)

The story of the manna and quail in the desert comes on the heels of the story of the bitter waters of Marah and Elim. In that provocative account, the Lord showed Moses a piece of wood, and when Moses threw the wood into the bitter water, the water that was once unpleasant became sweet, and the people could consume it and quench their thirst.

After they drank the water, Moses told them if they listened to the Lord, paid attention to Him, and did what was right in His eyes, God would not bring on them the diseases He brought on the people of Egypt (Genesis 15:22–26). As He intended at the waters of Marah and Elim, God's purpose was to heal His people. God takes great pleasure in His role as our Healer, and our access to His divine health plan is our loving faithfulness.

The context of following God is that He has plans to heal us along the way. Even when it comes to food, God intends for it to heal and not just simply meet the basic instinct of hunger.

Notice that the people complained that they were starving, but they did not look to the God who had just given them water for food, but they looked back to Egypt from the place in which God was trying to deliver them. They said, "There we sat around pots of meat and ate all the food we wanted" (v. 2). God was trying to deliver them from the bondage of Egypt, but the people craved the food of their captivity. Interestingly, people don't crave the food of their captivity— e.g., potato chips and ice cream—until they try to give them up and stop eating them; however, the devil doesn't let go of you without a fight. It's a struggle to break out of the bondage of bad eating, but keep clawing and scratching. Don't give up and throw in the towel. By the power of God, you are coming out. Remember: wanting to go back to an oppressive way of eating is fondly looking back to the place of your bondage.

To grasp fully the ramifications of how we develop the bad eating habits in our lives that lead to all kinds of health complications, recognize that eating is done in community. We are taught to like certain foods, we are taught to have certain cravings, and we are taught to think that what other people eat is strange. God's people said, "We sat . . . and ate." In other words, "This is how 'we' eat! Momma ate like this; daddy ate like this; we eat like this." But please look honestly at their lives. Was it a daily ritual of bad eating and then taking a handful of pills to counter the effect? You can't change what and who you came from, but you can change the way you eat.

For God to deliver us and change the bad food we desire, He often has to break us out of a cultivated mindset to crave what is bad for us. "Foods carry a power and an energy, and we must choose wisely what nourishes us and the world around us."[8] A willingness to expand your diet and taste is tantamount to going somewhere new and different, and once your thinking goes somewhere, it won't be long before you are headed somewhere new and different in life, so get ready.

> A WILLINGNESS TO EXPAND YOUR DIET AND TASTE IS TANTAMOUNT TO GOING SOMEWHERE NEW AND DIFFERENT, AND ONCE YOUR THINKING GOES SOMEWHERE, IT WON'T BE LONG BEFORE YOU ARE HEADED SOMEWHERE NEW AND DIFFERENT IN LIFE, SO GET READY.

---

[8] Harden, Neal. "Your Mission: Eat More Plants." *Dr. Oz The Good Life*. June 2017, p. 84.

God was trying to expand the people's tastes as He was leading them into His promises. All too often we have too narrow a view of food, which keeps us destined for the same health condition of the community that went before us and that suffered with any number of food related diseases—e.g., high blood pressure, high cholesterol, Type 2 diabetes, and aching joints. Expanding our culinary tastebuds opens us up to foods with the amazing ability to improve our overall wellness, energy level, state of mind, and our sense of being. How we feel about life and ourselves starts with what we eat. When we eat better, we will look and feel better.

As is familiar today, the people said of their time in Egypt we "ate all the food we wanted," but they said to Moses and Aaron, "You have brought us out into this desert to starve [us]." The one thing the enemy allowed them to do was overeat, and make no mistake about it, overeating is a trick of the enemy.

When I was younger, I used to think I was being helpful when I would try to tell people not to eat too much when I would see their plates piled high with food, but after getting told off a few times, I learned to leave people alone and just let them eat. People don't like limits on what they eat and how much they eat. It is not that overeaters don't know they are eating too much; they just don't want anyone to tell them.

The Bible says to "put a knife to your throat if you are given to gluttony" (Proverbs 23:2). Overeating is like killing yourself. The people were mad because God didn't want them to overeat. But He was doing it for their good—so they could have a totally blessed life with health and wellness.

I am sure you find it as interesting as I do that the people did not crave Egypt for the economic opportunity they had once enjoyed, and they did not crave Egypt because of the tranquil and lavish living conditions of the Egyptian suburbs, but they craved Egypt for the food. They craved the food of the place that was killing them. Don't crave that from which God is trying to deliver you. In the name of Jesus, ask God to take the taste of it from you right now. The Lord shows up that we might have life, and have it to the full (John 10:10).

Admittedly, some foods seem to almost call your name and will even go so far as to wake you up when you're asleep. One night chili dogs with light onions and mustard called my name. Well I jumped out of bed, went to the local grill and got two, and it seemed like a good idea at the time to wash those bad boys down with a blueberry milkshake. Needless to say in addition to feeling extremely guilty, I was so ashamed of myself the next morning. The sad part about it is I couldn't wait to go back and get two more. But later that day when I took off my shirt and looked in the mirror, there it was: Bondage staring me right in the face in the manifestation of a gut. Thank God I didn't go back to Egypt.

Don't go back to eating that from which the Lord is leading you away.

God's people most likely came out of Egypt overweight and in poor health, but they craved the very thing that put them in that condition: pots of meat. Studies have shown that "women who ate lots of vegetable protein—from seeds, beans, and soy—had a 30% reduced risk of heart disease and about 20% less chance of diabetes compared with those who got most of their protein from animal sources."[9] God was ensuring the

---

[9] Gold, Sunny Sea. "Your Mission: Eat More Plants." *Dr. Oz The Good Life*. June 2017, p. 82.

healing of his people as they followed Him in faithfulness in terms of how they ate. But they just didn't realize it.

The devil exercised power over them through their food. God had brought them out, but the devil was luring them back because of the food. Don't be enslaved by food. Demand in the name of Jesus to be set free.

So, God said to Moses, "I will rain down bread from heaven" (v. 4), and the test was to see if the people would follow God's instructions concerning the bread. It is important to point out that when the people said they were "starving," God did not give them pepperoni pizza, fried chicken, mashed potatoes and gravy, fried shrimp, or a hamburger and fries combo. He gave them bread, but before you judge the meager fare, hold on.

They were to eat the bread in the morning, and God would give them meat in the form of quail in the evening. Today we have become conditioned to think that we have to have meat for every meal. Sausage and eggs for breakfast, a hamburger and large fries for lunch, and roast beef and rice smothered in gravy for dinner. If God gave his people meat only in the evening, maybe there is a reason why. Speaking specifically of a love for meat, the Bible admonishes us not to "join those who drink too much wine or gorge themselves on meat, for drunkards and gluttons become poor and drowsiness clothes them in rags" (Proverbs 23:20–21). In actuality, some food experts today advise strongly in reserving meat for in the evening in that eating meat after dark helps to lose weight and restore health.[10]

---

[10] Gold, Sunny Sea. "Your Mission: Eat More Plants." *Dr. Oz The Good Life*. June 2017, p. 82.

The bread that God rained down from heaven was called manna, which means "what is it?" It was unlike anything the people had ever seen. When the people first encountered the bread, they had no idea what it was. However, when they experienced it, they said it looked like "coriander seed and tasted like wafers made with honey" (v. 31). The people didn't recognize the manna because they had only experienced food that was meant to keep them unhealthy and enslaved.

Not too long ago, my eldest son, whom I taught to drive and take care of a car, came in and presented me with an engine cleaner that he had just used in his car, and he told me how well it worked. I smiled, said, "Okay, cool," and sat it on the table. I thought to myself, "What does he know about cars? I taught him to drive." Well the car product sat right where he put it for weeks, and after a while, he said to me, "Dad, you're not going to use this are you?" I looked at him with that sheepish look we give people when we've been busted, and before I could answer, he said, "I'll take it back." I never thought too much about it, but a couple of days later I thought to myself, "I wonder if that stuff works?" So, I did some research and found out it is one of the best engine cleaners on the market today. I could have used something that would have really helped my car, but I was close-minded. A lot of people suffer bad health today because they are close-minded to God's instructions regarding food.

When the children of Israel experienced the manna, they recognized how good God's health plan is. Most of us need our mindset regarding food and our tastebuds set free from the bad habits of eating like the culture around us.

There is a reason why the psalmist wrote "O taste and see that the Lord is good" (Psalm 34:8). When we do things

God's way, and yes that even means when we eat His way, we experience His goodness. We look better, feel better, which will inevitably lead to living better.

Although no one has ever unlocked the mystery of the heavenly recipe of the manna, the Chef of heaven graciously allows us to share in the seasoning He used to flavor the wilderness cuisine: coriander seed and honey. The healing properties of the ingredients the Lord chose for this desert delicacy are a clear indication as to His purpose and intention for our food. (Note that other biblical herbs are also included in the following table.)

Herbs	Benefits	Preparation
Coriander Seed	• Facilitates beautiful skin and cures eczema, rashes, itchy skin • Helps against Type 2 diabetes • Stops hair from falling out and stimulates new hair growth • Lowers cholesterol • Strengthens immune system • Helps women maintain hormonal balance	• Dry-fry • Seasoning

Herbs	Benefits	Preparation
Cumin	• Aids in proper digestion • Fights against cancer cells • Builds iron/promotes energy • Strengthens immune system • May lower blood sugar • May lower cholesterol	• Lightly roasted • Spice
Mint	• Fights bacteria in the mouth • Promotes younger looking skin/stops acne • Fights cancer • Eliminates mucus from the airways • Helps stop flatulence • Relieves menstrual cramps • Prevents allergies	• Whole leaf • Chopped • Juice
Saffron	• Fights cancer • Treats memory loss and aids learning • Great sexual stimulant • Induces hair growth • Lowers cholesterol • Relieves stress	• Marinade • Baking

Herbs	Benefits	Preparation
Honey*	• Improves skin • Heals wounds and burns • Prevents cancer • Prevents heart disease • Reduces ulcers and gastrointestinal disorders • Increases athletic performance • Improves eyesight • Cures impotence/urinary tract disorders • Helps regulates blood sugar	• Raw • Topical treatment
Aloe	• Moisturizes hair and scalp • Strengthens immune system • Treats skin irritations and burns • Inhibits growth of harmful bacteria • Reduces dental plaque • Prevents wrinkles • Lowers blood sugar levels	• Topical treatment • Mouth rinse

Note that honey has a few more calories (21) per teaspoon than table sugar (16). However, current studies show honey "may not raise blood sugar as fast as other sweeteners, which is important because it's better for the body to have a slow, steady rise in blood sugar after eating rather than a dramatic spike."[11]

---

[11] Smith, Ian K. *Blast the Sugar Out! Lower Blood Sugar, Lose Weight, Live Better.* St. Martin's Press, 2017, p. 24.

ON-THE-WAY BLESSINGS

David, a man after God's own heart, realized something about the Lord when he said, "[He] forgives all your sins and heals all your diseases" (Psalm 103:3). If we just look at food from the spiritual aspect, we miss the fact that God was healing his people through the food they were eating as they were on the way to the promised land. Researchers today state definitely that certain foods "deliver extra-healthy versions of the energy molecules our bodies use as fuel. They also boost high levels of powerful phytonutrients (plant nutrients) that prevent all kinds of disease. The majority of medicines were [in fact] discovered in plants."[12] Diets with a lot of vegetables are really good for us. By eating a lot of vegetables, we're eating foods that are at the foundation of healing.

Eating pots full of meat is not good for anyone; eating too much red meat leads to all kinds of medical complications. The people needed to eat differently. The generation that came out of Egypt were undernourished and yet overfed as many of us are today. The type of food we eat matters. Don't crave food that keeps you in bondage. You can be free. Don't overeat. Mix into your diet healthy options. Eat food according to your faith, and you will see God heal your body.

> DON'T CRAVE FOOD THAT KEEPS YOU IN BONDAGE. YOU CAN BE FREE.

God was leading His people to the promised land, and on the way, He was healing their cancers, their diabetes, their high blood pressure, their cysts and tumors; He was healing their

---

[12] Grace, Tabitha. "Superfoods for Beginners." *The Power of Superfoods*. October 2017, p. 10.

infections and curing their wounds. On the way to what God had for them, they were being blessed. As you start trusting God with your food and how you eat, you're on the way to better. And while He's leading you there, He's healing you.

CLOSING PRAYER

Lord God my Healer, forgive me for the cravings that lead me to eat unhealthily. I surrender all to you now, and I come before You asking that You break every bad eating habit in my life—those that I learned from my community and those that are mine alone. Let food no longer be a driving force in my life, but let faithfulness be my motivation.

Amen.

Insights for Looking Better: _____

TASTE AND SEE

Insights for Feeling Better: _____

LOOK BETTER. FEEL BETTER. LIVE BETTER.

Insights for Living Better: _____

3

GOD'S FOOD AIN'T CHEAP

*"When I let go of what I am,
I become what I might be."*

—Lao Tzu

God's way of eating isn't cheap—it's rich. Let me explain.

Of all the amazing miracles performed by Jesus in the gospels of Matthew, Mark, Luke, and John, only one is recounted in all four: The miracle referred to as the Feeding of the Five Thousand. As such, it is completely understandable that such a feat would be found remarkable enough by all four writers to include it because there is no earthly way to explain it—no natural phenomenon bales out even the most ardent critic of the Bible. To feed five thousand men, and God only knows how many women and children there were, with only five loaves of bread and two fish is absolutely mind-boggling.

But what should be even more astounding to the person searching for God's secrets to His ordained health care plan is the fact that such a rich miracle was used involving what most people would consider to be cheap food, i.e., barley and two small fish—a boy's lunch.

Growing up as the oldest son of a single parent, life was not without its challenges. There was always a lot of love and plenty of laughter, but sometimes the laughter masked the pain and difficulty of just making it from one day to the next. Once when my mother was laid off, I found myself at eighteen the breadwinner for the family, but of course what I earned was never enough to get us completely through. As God would have it, a generous man in the neighborhood who worked on the local fishing dock and who admired me for trying to take care of my family would drop off a case of "borrowed" fish from the company every Friday in order that we might survive. At a time when everyone thought of steaks as "good eating," we were living off of the stollen fish provided by a good-hearted neighbor. Today I love to share with people my testimony about how God fed us the best when we didn't have any money at all, but we always thought we were eating "cheap food" because it was free. Today's prices of seafood back up my claim that we were eating the very best and didn't even realize it. Sometimes what appears cheap is actually God's best, but we don't always realize it. God's way of eating isn't cheap—it's rich.

> SOMETIMES WHAT APPEARS CHEAP IS ACTUALLY GOD'S BEST, BUT WE DON'T ALWAYS REALIZE IT.

LOOKING FOR A MIRACLE

Running after the types of foods the world values is extremely misleading, and because we think we are eating well when we are enjoying the high-caloric, processed fare of the culinary habits of the people around us, we completely dismiss the fact that God intends for food to heal us and not harm us. What looks good and desirable is not always good for us—just ask Eve. The world's way of eating will often set us up to be victims of the chronic diseases lurking at all of our genetic doors.

> Some time after this, Jesus crossed to the far shore of the Sea of Galilee (that is, the Sea of Tiberias), and a great crowd of people followed him because they saw the miraculous signs he had performed on the sick. Then Jesus went up on a mountainside and sat down with his disciples. The Jewish Passover Feast was near.
>
> When Jesus looked up and saw a great crowd coming toward him, he said to Philip, "Where shall we buy bread for these people to eat?" He asked this only to test him, for he already had in mind what he was going to do.
>
> Philip answered him, "Eight months' wages would not buy enough bread for each one to have a bite!"
>
> Another of his disciples, Andrew, Simon Peter's brother, spoke up, "Here is a boy with five small barley loaves and two small fish, but how far will they go among so many?"
>
> Jesus said, "Have the people sit down." There was plenty of grass in that place, and the men sat down,

about five thousand of them. Jesus then took the loaves, gave thanks, and distributed to those who were seated as much as they wanted. He did the same with the fish.

When they had all had enough to eat, he said to his disciples, "Gather the pieces that are left over. Let nothing be wasted."

So they gathered them and filled twelve baskets with the pieces of the five barley loaves left over by those who had eaten.

John 6:1–13 (NIV)

To start, given the incredible advances of modern medicine, the idea of looking to God for a miracle quite frankly makes many people feel a little silly, perhaps even somewhat naive and simple-minded. However, before there were all of the great health care options that are available today, people had to depend on the power of God to heal, deliver, and set them free. People looked to God for divine healing. Thus we can appreciate the excitement when the throngs of people who witnessed Jesus perform miracles on the sick proceeded to follow him across a sea and up on a mountainside.

The crowd wanted Jesus to do for them what they had seen him do for others. Where are you willing to follow Jesus for a miraculous healing of the maladies in your life? What is it that you really want the Lord to do for you?

For he satisfies the thirsty
and fills the hungry with good things.
—Psalm 107:9

It may seem silly and even cliché, but "Jesus Christ is the same yesterday and today and forever" (Hebrews 13:8). Follow him and he will heal you like he's healed countless others before you.

Both of my sons are living and breathing examples of God's power to heal. My youngest son was born with a degenerative tear duct that caused one of his eyes to clog with fluids that should have normally drained from his eye, but his eye would back up with fluid, and it would become infected. No matter how much medicine we put in his eye, the infection would always return, and the eye never healed.

Finally, the doctors told us the only way to ensure he would not grow up with a deformed eye was to have surgery. Well I made the decision to trust in God's power to heal him through prayer. Of course, there were some who resented my decision to trust in the power of God. The pressure of holding on to the promises of God got so bad that eventually I collapsed in tears for choosing to trust in the Lord's healing power.

One day when I couldn't take it anymore, my mother took my sons for a ride to give me a break, and while they were driving, someone in the car started screaming because out of nowhere, green puss gushed from my son's infected eye. The doctors couldn't explain it, but from that day forward my child never had another problem with that eye. Yes, make no mistake about it, God is a healer. Put your trust in Him today and believe He has a miracle just for you.

Looking at the miraculous story of the Feeding of the Five Thousand, don't miss the fact that when Jesus saw "a great crowd coming toward him," he was first concerned about what they were going to eat. Jesus knew they were following him to get healed of their diseases, but he did not address their medical needs until he addressed their nourishment need. There is an undeniable connection between what we eat and what we suffer. As such, researchers and nutrition experts are in agreement that if people really want to have and maintain a healthy brain and body, then having a complete diet, thereby getting all the needed nutrients, is of the utmost importance.

> THERE IS AN UNDENIABLE CONNECTION BETWEEN WHAT WE EAT AND WHAT WE SUFFER.

All too often we limit God's power to heal to the supernatural event of getting in a healing line in hopes that when it's our turn for the preacher to lay hands on us, the power of God will zap that malady right there and then. Some even help the preacher out with a courtesy fall. I once saw a woman peep out of one eye to see if it was okay to get up. Nevertheless, God is not limited to our limited understanding of healing—or even to our silly idiosyncrasies.

God can heal in any number of ways, such as using the food we eat. Jesus asked his disciple, "Where shall we buy bread for these people to eat?" In the same way Jesus is spiritually "the bread of life" that comes down from heaven which we can eat in faith and never die (John 5), Jesus is addressing the crowds' desire and need for bodily healing through the bread that they eat.

IN JESUS' HANDS

First, when Jesus' disciples presented him with a solution to the dilemma of feeding the great crowd, it was a young lad's lunch of "five small barley loaves and two small fish." Indeed, a small answer for a huge problem. However, God never overlooks what seems inconsequential. What is small in our hands is mighty when put in God's hands. Whole grains, vegetables and nuts are cheap and easily overlooked, but put them in the Lord's hands and anticipate the supernatural.

I heard a memorable story once about what happens when we put our needs and issues in God's hands. A young seminarian was invited to a remote area of the country to hold a revival, and after nights of skillful preaching, the young man became the talk of the town. One evening after a particularly rousing service, an apparent lay minister humbly approached the young seminary student and asked if he could maybe come and say a few words one day at his church.

The seminary student readily agreed, and a few weeks later met the older man at the church where he had been invited. When he arrived he was shocked at how beautiful the church was, especially for such an out-of-the-way place, so excitedly the young man asked if he could meet the pastor of such a "fine edifice." The old lay minister looked at the youngster, shyly smiled, and said, "I'm the pastor." The seminarian was shocked and a little embarrassed. The older preacher again smiled, looked down, and said, "Sometimes God can strike a mighty straight blow when you put a crooked stick in His hands."

GOD'S FOOD AIN'T CHEAP

*The eyes of all look to you,
and you give them their food at
the proper time.
You open your hand
and satisfy the desires of every living thing.*
—Psalm 145:15–16

> PUT YOUR EATING HABITS IN GOD'S HANDS, TRUST HIM TO HEAL YOUR BODY, AND HE WILL DO IT FOR YOU. JUST BELIEVE.

Put your eating habits in God's hands, trust Him to heal your body, and He will do it for you. Just believe.

It is only in the gospel of John that the type of loaves presented to Jesus is mentioned. Barley is considered the food of the poor. Yet, God has more than once used this seemingly meager, inconsequential food to do great things. Through the word of the Lord, the prophet Elisha once took twenty loaves of barley bread from a single faithful and fed a hundred hungry men, having had some bread left over. If you have the faith, God has the power in His hands.

The bread was a gift to the prophet from a faithful servant for the sustenance of the man of God, and Elisha performed a miracle with it (2 Kings 4:42–44).

When barley bread is put in Jesus' hands by faith, he again performs a mighty miracle with it. In faith, God takes the least to do the greatest. There is a great miracle for God's people when barley bread is received and eaten in faith. The apostle Paul reminds us that God chooses the "lowly things of this world and the despised things—and the things that are not—to nullify the things that are" (1 Corinthians 1:28). You can nullify the diseases in your body by eating the food which the Lord chooses to perform miracles. Plant-based eating has what food experts and researchers call miraculous benefits. Swapping beans and fruits for meats is introducing your body to all kinds of healthy minerals and substances. In fact, plants are packed with the types of nutrients that "help you live better and longer, without getting afflicted by the chronic diseases that drag us all down."[13] There is a miracle waiting to happen in your life when you eat in faith the food the Lord chooses.

Jesus "took the loaves, gave thanks, and distributed to those who were seated as much as they wanted." Before he distributed the loaves to the men who were seated, Jesus directed his disciples to instruct the nearly five thousand men who had followed him across the sea and up the rocky mountainside to be seated in the grass. Jesus did not give the miracle bread to anyone who was not seated, but only to those who had followed the disciples' instructions.

Don't come as far as you have and miss your blessing because you refuse to humble yourself in the presence of the Lord and eat the humble food he has used so powerfully in the past to heal others. A Syrian general by the name of Naaman, at the behest of his attendants, had to humble himself, but when he did, and he dipped in the dirty water he thought he was too good for, God released a powerful anointing and healed his diseased body of leprosy right there and then (2 Kings 5:13). Whatever the Lord wants you to do, do it! Your healing is connected to your faithfulness.

> DON'T COME AS FAR AS YOU HAVE AND MISS YOUR BLESSING BECAUSE YOU REFUSE TO HUMBLE YOURSELF IN THE PRESENCE OF THE LORD AND EAT THE HUMBLE FOOD HE HAS USED SO POWERFULLY IN THE PAST TO HEAL OTHERS.

---

[13] Gold, Sunny Sea. "Your Mission: Eat More Plants." *Dr. Oz The Good Life.* June 2017, p. 85.

Interestingly, Jesus' giving of thanks and distributing the bread foreshadows the ritual of the Lord's Supper. If barley bread is good enough for the Lord's food, it should be good enough for those of us seeking the Lord's miraculous healing power to touch our lives.

There are some incredible nutritional facts of whole grain of which we all need to be reminded.

Whole Grain	Benefits	Preparation
Barley	• Maintains a healthy colon • Fights toxins • Ensures strong bones • Promotes youthful appearance of skin • Helps control cholesterol • Lowers blood sugar • Prevents cancer	• Boil • Bake
Wheat*	• Prevents Type 2 diabetes • Reduces blood estrogen • Fights breast cancer • Fights heart disease • Reduces inflammation	• Bake • Boil

Whole Grain	Benefits	Preparation
Sorghum	• Reduces risk of cancer • Controls diabetes • Boosts energy • Prevents arthritis • Fights anemia	• Toasted • Popped • Baked
Oats	• Lowers cholesterol • Lowers blood sugar • Beautifies skin • Lowers blood pressure • Strengthens immune system	• Topical treatment • Baking • Smoothies
Maize (Corn)	• Fights tumors • Fights heart disease • Lowers cholesterol • Lowers blood pressure • Promotes healthy skin • Strengthens immune system • Lowers blood sugar	• Steam • Bake • Grill
Rice	• Lowers blood pressure • Prevents cancer (i.e., brown rice) • Promotes healthy skin • Lowers cholesterol • Fights heart disease	• Steam • Topical treatment • Rice water

* *Always check with a physician before consuming large amounts of wheat.*

As much as Jesus' miracle of the Feeding of the Five Thousand is a prophetic statement of who he is, his decision to use barley bread when the people were looking for a miracle is indicative of a food selected by God to heal His people. Although the fish put at Jesus' disposal was part of the youth's fare, the fish in the story seems to be an afterthought of sorts. Notice that when the festal occasion was over, only the pieces of bread that were left over were "gathered" so that they would not be wasted, indicating that the barley bread has miracle healing power for God's people extending well into the future. The Lord is telling us that in faith it still has healing power.

Nevertheless, the benefits of a diet that includes fish should be expressly mentioned as we have seen throughout scripture that Jesus more than once fed his disciples with fish. More specifically, "The American Heart Association recommends two servings of fatty fish, like tuna or salmon, a week for their abundant omega-3 fatty acids, which have been linked to improving memory function and promoting healthy skin."[14] Thus, the protein provided by fish and other quality food sources is extremely important. As people age, they need more protein. A diet packed with high-quality proteins supplies the body with energy as it maintains and repairs muscles.[15]

---

[14] Friedlander, Steven, Editor-in-Chief. "The Power of Protein." *100 Ways to Live to 100: Expert Advice for a Longer Life*. July 2017, p. 74.

[15] Gold, Sunny Sea. "Your Mission: Eat More Plants." *Dr. Oz The Good Life*. June 2017, p. 93.

Fish	Benefits	Preparation
Salmon	• Lowers blood pressure • Reduces inflammation • Promotes skin health • Maintains muscle strength • Produces energy • Fights heart disease • Fights cancer	• Bake • Grill • Sauté
Mackerel	• Fights heart disease • Produces energy • Lowers cholesterol • Prevents arthritis • Prevents mental illness • Fights cancer	• Bake • Grill • Sauté
Sardines	• Prevents cancer • Promotes bone health • Beautifies skin • Promotes hair growth • Lowers cholesterol • Lowers blood pressure	• Canned • Baked • Grilled

CLOSING PRAYER

Lord Jesus, all creation looks to You for food—the birds of the air, the beasts of the field, the fish of the sea, and I, Your child. I desire what You provide for my life, for from Your hands come healing and restoration. When you feed me, I will enjoy rich fare according to Your will. In faith, I put my eating habits in Your hands that miraculous healing may be mine.

Amen.

Insights for Looking Better: _____

GOD'S FOOD AIN'T CHEAP

Insights for Feeling Better:

LOOK BETTER. FEEL BETTER. LIVE BETTER.

Insights for Living Better: _____

4

FELLOWSHIP OF A MIRACLE

"The first step toward success is taken when you refuse to be a captive of the environment in which you first find yourself."

—Mark Caine

Food is ultimately intended for fellowship. To ignore the communal aspect of food is to miss the substitutionary significance God intends when we sit down to eat. Besides food's purpose of satisfying our basic instinct of hunger, food is also intended to maintain the perfection of God's creation as well as heal the imperfections resulting when our inclinations and proclivities take us too far away from the presence and will of God. In the same way eating bad food takes us away from the well-being God intended, eating how and what God desires ushers us back into the divine image we were meant to exhibit.

When the apostle Paul says, "Everything is permissible—but not everything is beneficial" (1 Corinthians 10:23), his context is food and fellowship. If we should be concerned about the good of others when we eat, then it only stands to reason that God is also concerned about our well-being when we eat in fellowship with Him. Eating involves the good of others. When we eat, God wants our good to come from it.

A RENEWED IMAGE

> If someone's offering is a fellowship offering, and he offers an animal from the herd, whether male or female, he is to present before the Lord an animal without defect. He is to lay his hand on the head of his offering and slaughter it at the entrance to the Tent of Meeting. Then Aaron's sons the priests shall sprinkle the blood against the altar on all sides.
>
> Leviticus 3:1–2 (NIV)

The reason the Israelites were instructed to get "an animal without defect" for a fellowship offering was because when the offerer laid hands on the head of the creature, the purity of the unblemished animal was attributed to the marred worshiper desperately seeking relief and restoration, for "He is to lay his hand on the head of his offering." As a symbolic act of identification, the worshipper laid his hand on the animal and looked at the unblemished beast and saw the qualities he would acquire. When you identify with

> WHEN YOU IDENTIFY WITH THE FOOD YOU'RE GOING TO EAT, YOU'RE INVITING THE BENEFITS OF THE MEAL INTO YOUR LIFE.

the food you're going to eat, you're inviting the benefits of the meal into your life. Identify with the miracle in your food, and you're inviting that miracle, i.e., lower cholesterol, lower blood pressure, healthy hair, healthy bones, strengthened immune system, energy, etc. into your life. Food has an incalculable value when it is enjoyed in an attitude of fellowship with the Lord. Don't just eat to eat; rather, eat to worship in fellowship with God, receiving the goodness and healing power from food the way food is intended to do.

I will satisfy the priests with abundance, and my people will be filled with my bounty.
—JEREMIAH 31:14

Food enjoyed as part of fellowship is an extension of the concept of the Hebrew word *shalom*, which means wholeness and peace. Partaking of food when the Lord is involved in it is tantamount to receiving what is His and God receiving what is yours. To be sure, the only offering that the worshipper could partake of was the fellowship offering because God knows that when we sit down to eat with Him, we are brought back into wholeness.

But you have to want to be whole. In the same way no one can make you stop ordering extra large fries every time you go to a restaurant or stop you from sneaking to the doughnut shop at night, you have to want wholeness. Wholeness and inner peace don't come out of compulsion or duress. You have to desire it like the apostle Matthew desired a change for his life. I can imagine when Jesus extended to him the chance for a change, the beleaguered Israelite leaped from the table he was at in order to sit at the table with the Lord. It's time for a glorious change in your life.

CHANGE OF ATTITUDE

The association of food, fellowship, and healing are no where better illustrated than in the account of the calling of Matthew the tax collector:

> As Jesus went from there, he saw a man named Matthew sitting at the tax collector's booth. "Follow me," he told him, and Matthew got up and followed him.
>
> While Jesus was having dinner at Matthew's house, many tax collectors and "sinners" came and ate with him and his disciples. When the Pharisees saw this,

they asked his disciples, "Why does your teacher eat with tax collectors and 'sinners'?"

On hearing this, Jesus said, "It is not the healthy who need a doctor, but the sick. But go and learn what this mean: 'I desire mercy, not sacrifice.' For I have not come to call the righteous, but sinners."

Matthew 9:9–13 (NIV)

After calling Matthew from a tax collector's table, Jesus later dined with him, where he and his disciples were joined by other tax collectors and people simply designated as "sinners." Upon seeing Jesus comfortably dine with such notorious guests, the local Pharisees questioned Jesus' actions, "Why does your teacher eat with tax collectors and 'sinners'?" to which he replied, 'It is not the healthy who need a doctor, but the sick.'" Although Matthew was loathed, Jesus ate with him in order to heal him. How family and coworkers might think of you won't stop the Lord from fellowshipping with you.

Jesus didn't ask Matthew to get in a healing line, and he didn't ask him to run around the church three times; to heal him, the Lord sat down at the table with him and ate with him. When you sit down to eat, invite Jesus to sit down with you, and he will.

> JESUS DIDN'T ASK MATTHEW TO GET IN A HEALING LINE, AND HE DIDN'T ASK HIM TO RUN AROUND THE CHURCH THREE TIMES; TO HEAL HIM, THE LORD SAT DOWN AT THE TABLE WITH HIM AND ATE WITH HIM.

Although tax collectors were a part of society, most Jews avoided people like Matthew because association with him and his kind could negatively affect one's reputation. Even today, people viewed as socially unacceptable are avoided. People who do not fit, who do not look like us, and who embarrass us are often left out. But anyone who wants to leave an unpleasant lifestyle behind such as the sick who look to be healed will find that fellowship with Jesus is the cure.

To dine with someone is significant because of the symbolic nature of the gesture. To dine with someone is to accept him. Jesus accepted Matthew, and the Lord accepts you. Regardless of what you've done, and despite the mistakes in life you may have made, the Lord accepts you.

When Jesus told the shamed and scorned Matthew to "Follow me," and the newly minted disciple proceeded to get up and follow him, we all can smile in reflection and relate to this type of deliverance because it is comforting to think that God will lead us away from what has caused us trouble and defeat all of our lives. We all would like God to take us by the hand and just triumphantly walk us away from our problems and issues. But notice that Jesus actually did the exact opposite. He didn't lead Matthew away from his problems; rather, he led him back to the root of his issues, for "[w]hile Jesus was having dinner at Matthew's house" indicates that Jesus had to heal him at the table before he could use him, and his healing would take place with food.

Diets and eating practices have gotten so far away from what God intended for His people that we all need to be taken back to what God actually intended for food. In order to receive the miracle of healing in food, we all need to examine our attitude as to how we think of food. Jesus took the disciple from a cursed table to a blessed table. When Jesus is at the table with you, it is a place of blessings and healing.

If you want to be what you know God always intended for you to be, look at your table differently. The Pharisees looked at the table Jesus and Matthew were sitting at, but they never saw what the Lord was doing at the table, "Why does your teacher eat with tax collectors and 'sinners'?" People will look at you and criticize you for thinking a new way about your food and thus eating a new way, but Jesus will be there with you, healing you. People will try to get you to eat what you don't want to eat, and they will try to force upon you their weaknesses. But tell them your doctor, i.e., the One who has never lost a patient, said not to eat it.

> IF YOU WANT TO BE WHAT YOU KNOW GOD ALWAYS INTENDED FOR YOU TO BE, LOOK AT YOUR TABLE DIFFERENTLY.

Interestingly, it should be observed that when Matthew invited Christ into his home to dine, he, too, invited his disciples. In other words, when you welcome Jesus to fellowship with you when you are eating food, you must likewise receive all that belongs to him to eat with you also. In this light, all that is yours is also welcome to dine as was the case with Matthew—his friends, his associates, his embarrassments—for "[w]hen Jesus was having dinner at Matthew's house, many tax collectors and 'sinners' came and ate with him and his disciples." When you open your heart to Jesus to sit and fellowship with you, all your food issues and proclivities are welcome: overeating is welcome, food addiction is welcome, eating disorders are welcome, weakness is welcome, and cravings are welcome.

Recently, I was traveling out of town to visit a family that had just lost a loved one. When I got to the home, people and food were everywhere, and before I could get in the door to greet everyone, someone yelled, "Rev., you want something to eat?" Then, before I could politely decline, someone else blurted out, "Fix him something to eat," so I politely ate instead. My plate was full of fried chicken, as you might have guessed, coleslaw and hush puppies. The chicken was good, but I keep noticing the grease in the plate and thought to myself, "Lord, help me."

On the way home, I was casually driving along a dark road when I rode by a billboard that made me look twice. The handsome sign read, "MEAT INTERRUPTS YOUR SEX LIFE. Meat and dairy clog your arteries and can lead to erectile dysfunction."[16] Well I got out of my car, took a picture, and said to myself, "Lord, You heard my cry. Now please heal my body of all that greasy chicken."

What really grabbed my attention about the billboard was that beside the words was a picture of a couple, who was lying in bed, obviously troubled by their copulatory dysfunction. She was on her back, looking frustratedly off to the left, and he was turned on his side, looking dejectedly off to the right. But lying in the middle of them was a pig, and that little dirty, God-prohibited rascal was sleeping like a baby.

In the healing presence of the Lord, what you desperately want God to do for you is welcome. God will get the interruptions out of your life, out of your marriage, and out of your performance if you will invite him to dine with you. There is a miracle waiting to happen in your life through table fellowship with the Lord. Don't let what you don't want in your life interrupt what you do want in your life. Let God change your attitude about what you eat.

---

[16] *PeTA* Billboard, Fayetteville, NC. 2017.

*The Lord will reply to them:
"I am sending you grain, new wine
and oil,
enough to satisfy you fully;
never again will I make you
an object of scorn to the nations."*
—Joel 2:19

Don't be shy about that from which you want to be delivered, and invite all your food issues and proclivities to the table with the Doctor of your soul.

Given the communal appearance of the dinner at Matthew's house—involving a meal shared with others, it is highly probable that the beleaguered disciple hosted a fellowship meal, which had specific food items, such as animals from the herd or the flock, and different cakes of bread (see Chapter 3) made without yeast and mixed with oil.

Meats	Benefits	Preparation
Beef (grass-fed)*	• Reduces risk of cancer • Reduces risk of heart disease • Controls heart disease • Reduces risk of food poisoning	• Grill • Sauté • Bake
Lamb (grass-fed)*	• Prevents cancer • Prevents obesity • Lowers cholesterol • Promotes skin health • Maintains bone health	• Grill • Sauté • Bake
Deer*	• Helps control blood sugar • Builds muscle • Enhances immune system • Helps control cholesterol	• Grill • Sauté • Bake

Consume in moderation.

As discussed throughout this book, God uses very little meat in the nourishing and healing of His people when food is His modus operandi. Against this backdrop, many experts who espouse plant-based diets for healthy eating habits admonish those looking for dietary answers to health and wholeness to steer clear of a lot of red meat. Researchers now, however, are finding that grass-fed meat, as opposed to grain-fed and soy-fed meat, is actually health-promoting because the meat is leaner and doesn't do as much harm to the body. Still and all, the world's healthiest people have diets built around plants rather than meat. Notwithstanding, people desiring the taste of red meat will find that today's grass-fed meat is leaner and thus healthier, which has to have been the case in Jesus' time given the fact current farming methods had yet to be developed and put into operation.

For the guests dining at Matthew's house when Jesus was the guest of honor, they became intimate with the Lord, and the Pharisees' negative question couldn't stop the life-changing relationship but rather highlighted the type of renewal and restoration God wants all of us to have with him as we eat more faithfully. When we eat the way God wants us to eat, He adopts a new and exciting role in our lives: divine healer. Eating with Jesus means more than just eating a meal; it means restoration and renewal. Shutting it down, Jesus declared, "It is not the healthy who need a doctor, but the sick," affirming that through table fellowship with him, he was going to heal Matthew with acceptance and mercy.

When you sit down to eat, start by inviting Jesus to dine with you. What happens next is a life-changing fellowship between you and the Lord.

CLOSING PRAYER

Lord God, You came in Your Son Jesus that I might have fellowship with You. Don't leave me at a table that is destroying me, but call me to eat in Your merciful and healing presence, that in the food I eat, I may more faithfully identify with You, receiving what is Yours, that wholeness and inner peace may become mine. Remove from me, I pray, all manner of illness and disease.

Amen.

Insights for Looking Better: _____

_____
_____
_____
_____
_____
_____
_____
_____
_____
_____
_____
_____
_____
_____

Insights for Feeling Better:

LOOK BETTER. FEEL BETTER. LIVE BETTER.

Insights for Living Better: _____

5

"ALMOST, NOT YET"

"The only limit to the height of your achievements is the reach of your dreams and your willingness to work hard for them."
—Michelle Obama

One of my fondest, and at the same time most frustrating, childhood memories of family meals is remembering smelling what was cooking in the kitchen but having to wait for it to be ready. Like most people tantalized by the smell of something good being prepared and at the same time being frustrated with the endless anguish of wondering when it would ever be ready, I would run to the kitchen every five minutes or so to ask, "Ma, is it ready yet?" only to hear my mother's canned reply, "Almost, not yet." Well to let her know how displeased I was, I'd poke my lips out, sigh as deeply as I could, and stomp out of the kitchen. I don't think it made her cook any faster, but it certainly made me feel better (at least I thought so).

Waiting for something good to come to you can seem like an eternity, especially when what you're waiting for is out of your control. However, as with the metaphorical woman waiting to give birth in Jesus' comforting words to his disciples as he was preparing them for his departure, if we hold on and don't give up, our grief and pain does turn to joy (John 16:21). Nevertheless, sometimes waiting brings certain undeniable biological changes into our lives, such as lost friendships, graying hair, gaining weight, losing strength, and the prospect of giving up on our dreams.

If you are willing and obedient,

you will eat the best from the land.

—Isaiah 1:19

But the question is this: if God has asked you to wait while He is preparing your miracle, how does he intend to keep you strong and vibrant while you're waiting so that when the answer to your prayer does come, you have the strength to enjoy it?

STRENGTH WHILE YOU WAIT

The trek from Egypt to the promised land was arduous and excruciatingly difficult. So much so that only two people who came out of the bondage of Egypt, Joshua and Caleb, actually entered into the land of Canaan, also known to them as the promised land. People lost their faith, rebelled against God, got weak, and died—ultimately without ever entering into God's promises. A journey, that started out with such enthusiasm and great expectation, should have taken only eleven days; it ended up taking forty years (Deuteronomy 1:2). For most of us, when we finally get our minds made up that we are going to accomplish something epic, we usually see it happening within a reasonable amount of time, and we have no idea how long it can actually take.

> Now the men of Judah approached Joshua at Gilgal, and Caleb son of Jephunneh the Kenizzite said to him, "You know what the Lord said to Moses the man of God at Kadesh Barnea about you and me. I was forty years old when Moses the servant of the Lord sent me from Kadesh Barnea to explore the land. And I brought him back a report according to my convictions, but my brothers who went up with me made the hearts of the people melt with fear. I,

however, followed the Lord my God wholeheartedly. So on that day Moses swore to me, "The land on which your feet have walked will be your inheritance and that of your children forever, because you have followed the Lord my God wholeheartedly."

Now then, just as the Lord promised, he has kept me alive for forty-five years since the time he said this to Moses, while Israel moved about in the desert. So here I am today, eighty-five years old! I am still as strong today as the day Moses sent me out; I'm just as vigorous to go out to battle now as I was then. Now give me this hill country that the Lord promised me that day.

Joshua 14:6–12 (NIV)

Sometimes our greatest blessings come later in life. Caleb was eighty-five when he stepped forward and laid claim on what God had promised him forty-five years earlier. Most people at eighty-five are waiting to transition. They feel their lives are over; they don't have the energy to attempt anything new; they think their best years are behind them. Believe it or not, "recent studies show strong correlation between depression, dementia and other brain-based illnesses and what we eat. Add this data to the modern discovery that brains actually continue growing into adulthood, and the conclusions are startling. The nutrients many people are missing are the most important to brain health."[17] Advanced years don't mean new and exciting things in our lives are over. If we change our thinking about aging and food, we'd see that God has so much more for us than our numbers actually indicate.

---

[17] Grace, Tabitha. "You Are What You Eat." *The Power of Superfoods*. October 2017, p. 13.

To the contrary, the Bible is full of geriatric giants of the faith—people who trusted God into the later years of life: Abraham and Sarah had their first baby at one hundred and ninety years old, respectively (Genesis 17:17); Moses was eighty when God had finished preparing him and started using him in his life's work (Exodus 7:7); even Elizabeth, Mary's relative, was blessed "in her old age" to conceive and give birth to John the Baptist (Luke 1:36). For God, old age is fertile ground for miracles. Don't ever stop thinking that God is going to do something great in your life. Don't ever give up the hope that your season is about to come. If you ever give up, then you stop being ready and excited about what's being prepared just for you. You stop running to Him. You stop asking Him when will it be ready. As we see with Caleb, God is keeping you alive and allowing you to wander in the desert of hope and trust in His promises just so you can step forward in the company of men and claim what everyone knows you've been waiting for—to the glory of God.

> DON'T EVER STOP THINKING THAT GOD IS GOING TO DO SOMETHING GREAT IN YOUR LIFE. DON'T EVER GIVE UP THE HOPE THAT YOUR SEASON IS ABOUT TO COME.

The dilemma for us today is that Caleb declared he was "still as strong" at eighty-five as he was "the day Moses sent [him] out." Even more audaciously, he insisted he was just "as vigorous to go out to battle" at eighty-five as he was when he was forty. How in the world could that be? How can an eighty-five-year-old man be just as "vigorous" as a forty-year-old man? Unlike Caleb, more than 70 percent of the people in the world today are under nourished, i.e., not getting the nutrients they need for proper health, leading to many kinds of chronic diseases and robbing them of physical fitness and overall wellness. The result is that when most of God's people get old, instead of being valiant warriors for the kingdom, they are not ready or willing to take on anything new in life; rather, they start looking around for Father Time to tap them on the shoulder to say, "Let's go home."

When my grandmother was in her eighties, shortly before she passed away, I remember her telling me, "Derrick, I'm just tired. I'm ready to go home." I pleaded with her not to say that, but that's just how she felt. Many people when they get to a certain point in life just don't have the energy to go on. But not Caleb. Why?

Any understanding of the senior citizen superstar must go back to the moment that singled him out as a giant of the faith. At the Lord's command, Moses had to select a leader from each of the twelve tribes of Israel to form a cohort that would go and spy out the land of Canaan. Caleb was selected from the tribe of Judah, which is in itself interesting because Caleb was not a native Israelite. Yet, his selection just goes to show that God honors faithfulness over kinship. You don't have to depend upon, or be limited to, human relationships in order to get ahead and prosper in God's kingdom, just be faithful in God's eyes.

So, Moses sent the spies to Canaan on a reconnoissance mission to find out everything they could about the land: whether it had good soil or bad soil, walled or unwalled cities, strong or weak people, wooded or grasslands, and if the fruit was good or basic. Specifically, the last thing Moses told the men was to do their "best to bring back some of the fruit of the land" (Numbers 13:20). As such, the spies explored the land for forty days, wand when they got to the Valley of

Eshcol, along with some pomegranates and figs, they cut off a cluster of grapes that was so large and heavy two men had to carry it on a pole in order to get it back to Moses.

The fruit of the land was indicative of the condition of the land; if the fruit was good, then the land, too, had to be good. Likewise, the fruit was indicative of the stature of the people. That is, if the people ate good fruit, they would be a mighty people, confirmed by the fact "the descendants of Anak," who were both powerful and of great size, lived there (Numbers 13:28).

Moses, it should be pointed out, wanted to see the food because if he could see the food, then he could understand the condition of the people and the state of their land. The food you eat tells the world all about you, and when faith is mixed with the right food, food is indicative of destiny.

At the end of the time set by the king to bring them in,

the chief official presented them to Nebuchadnezzar.

The king talked with them, and he found none equal to Daniel, Hananiah, Mishael and Azariah; so they entered the king's service.

In every matter of wisdom and understanding about which

the king questioned them, he found them ten times better than all the magicians and enchanters in his whole kingdom.

—Daniel 1:18–20

Eating more faithfully involves eating more healthy foods, such as vegetables and fruits, which studies show leads to more enjoyment in life and more longevity. Diets built around plants produce the happiest and healthiest people, with the God-intended benefit of reducing blood pressure, promoting an increased metabolic rate, hormone balance, and improving cholesterol. When you look and feel better, you are more confident and assertive—and people will notice.

When Moses told the spies to bring back some fruit, he wanted them to see what they would be eating if they trusted in God. Thus, if God gave it to them to eat, then He intended for them to benefit from it.

The ten spies who were not allowed to enter the promised land appreciated the size of the food, but they did not mix their faith with the food. Caleb mixed his faith with the food, and God gave him everything associated with the food: the land, the health, the longevity. Start mixing your faith with your food, and start right away.

> CALEB MIXED HIS FAITH WITH THE FOOD, AND GOD GAVE HIM EVERYTHING ASSOCIATED WITH THE FOOD: THE LAND, THE HEALTH, THE LONGEVITY.

At eighty-five, Caleb was living according to what God said he could have. He believed he could have the land that produced the grapes, and God gave him the benefits of the fruit he carried in faith: good health, strength, and vigor. Believe you can have what God says you can have, and you will see it manifest in your life.

Here are some of the amazing benefits of the fruit from the promised land Caleb carried back to the camp in faith.

(Anti-Aging) Fruit	Benefits	Preparation
Grapes*	• Fights asthma • Prevents Acne • Strengthens bones and prevents osteoporosis • Good for eye health • Helps flatten the stomach • Reduces the risks of heart attacks • Helps brain functions • Cures migraines • Prevents fatigue • Lowers cholesterol levels • Helps prevent breast cancer	• Fresh • Dried • Juice
Pomegranates	• Fights cancer • Decreases risk of strokes and heart attacks • Reduces anemia • Cures erectile dysfunction • Fights cancer • Lowers blood pressure • Fights joint pain • Improves memory	• Deseed • Juice

(Anti-Aging) Fruit	Benefits	Preparation
Figs	• Helps with sexual vitality • Helps control Type 2 diabetes • Strengthens bones • Stimulates hair growth • Beautifies the skin • Helps prevent heart attack • Protects from cancer	• Fresh • Dried • Poached

* *Grapes are extremely high in natural sugar, so it is recommended that they be consumed in moderation.*

BLESSED FOOD

Although we are never told when the great general for the Lord passed away, we do know that at eighty-five Caleb was still going strong, living to take more land from the enemy and to give his daughter's hand in marriage. Nevertheless, we should not count it strange that his later years were just as vivacious as his younger years. God specifically says, "Worship the Lord your God, and his blessing will be on your food and water. I will take away sickness from among you, and none will miscarry or be barren in your land. I will give you a full life span" (Exodus 23:25–26). The one thing we do know about Caleb is that he worshipped God "wholeheartedly." As a result, God blessed the food he ate and took disease and sickness from his life. Can you imagine the wonder in the eyes of the younger people around Caleb who witnessed him coming out of the desert with more optimism and vigor than men half his age? Caleb's old age wasn't marred by the dusty chronic diseases of the unfaithful, but it represented the blessedness and favor that comes with putting faith in God. What Caleb went through surviving the wilderness didn't rob him of his outlook and hope; rather, what he experienced and went through in life strengthened and emboldened his outlook.

So whether you eat or drink or whatever you do,

do it all for the glory of God.
—1 Corinthians 10:31

When Caleb ate in faith his figs, pomegranates, and grapes under the heavens, God allowed the benefits of his food to infuse him with power and might. When faith in God is mixed with the food we eat, God puts healing power in our food to heal us and give us a long, healthy life.

God is preparing something special for you. While you're waiting and being tantalized with expectation, don't get frustrated, poke your lips out, stomp away, and give up. Keep yourself strong in faith and body by eating God's way, and let God bless your food, and you will receive the benefits of His promise.

CLOSING PRAYER

Lord of heaven and all the earth, bless all that I eat as I eat in wholehearted faithfulness to you. Instead of allowing me to lose strength while I wait, Dear Lord, let what I eat increase my strength and outlook on life. I stand on the promises You have for my life, and by faith I believe I will eat the fruit of the land.

Amen.

LOOK BETTER. FEEL BETTER. LIVE BETTER.

Insights for Looking Better: _____

"ALMOST, NOT YET"

Insights for Feeling Better: _____

LOOK BETTER. FEEL BETTER. LIVE BETTER.

Insights for Living Better:

6

THE CHILDREN'S CRUMBS

"Go out on a limb. That's where the fruit is."
—Jimmy Carter

Good food is always appreciated, e.g., when we're trying to get to know people with whom we work. Food facilitates friendship and all manner of conversation; when we celebrate a loved one's birthday, we often do it around festive food; when our hearts are sad and have been broken, food makes us feel better; when we've come through a storm, food reassures us that everything is going to be all right. Indeed, food soothes and helps us to cope with life. As it were, we all have deep needs that food seems to settle and heal beyond the simple need to eat, so in God's infinite wisdom, food has to be understood and enjoyed as well as be employed strategically.

Despite being a gift, life is full of ups and downs and the ebb and flow of circumstances. If we aren't careful, life can drain us of our strength and energy to make it from one day to the next. Have you ever noticed that when you're really stressed and experiencing a particularly trying time, you eat more? Thus what you eat in relation to what you're going through is critical. If we indeed need food in coping with life's turbulence, then doesn't it make sense to have that food which meets the need?

DON'T FORGET THE OIL

The story of the sinful woman who anointed Jesus' feet while he dined at Simon's house is particularly engaging for someone having the right food to meet the need.

> Jesus answered him, "Simon, I have something to tell you."
>
> "Tell me, teacher," he said.
>
> "Two men owed money to a certain moneylender. One owed him five hundred denarii, and the other fifty. Neither of them had the money to pay him back, so he canceled the debts of both. Now which of them will love him more?"
>
> Simon replied, "I suppose the one who had the bigger debt canceled."
>
> "You have judged correctly," Jesus said.
>
> Then he turned toward the woman and said to Simon, "Do you see this woman? I came into your house. You did not give me any water for my feet, but

she wet my feet with her tears and wiped them with her hair. You did not give me a kiss, but this woman, from the time I entered, has not stopped kissing my feet. You did not put oil on my head, but she has poured perfume on my feet. Therefore, I tell you, her many sins have been forgiven—for she loved much. But he who has been forgiven little loves little."

Luke 7:40–48 (NIV)

Jesus had been invited to dinner, and the man who invited him apparently had plenty of food with which to entertain his guests, but he had failed to supply any oil. A woman with a seedy past, however, came to the dinner also (perhaps uninvited), but she brought oil—expensive oil. After she washed Jesus' feet with her tears, she proceeded to anoint them with the oil, to which she brought upon Jesus secret criticism by the host of the dinner for the type of life she had lived.

To show the man how wrong his thinking about him and the woman was, Jesus told a parable about a creditor who had two debtors; one owed a lot, and the other owed a little. Since neither could repay their debt, the creditor forgave them both. Then Jesus asked the judgmental patron, who do you think will love the creditor more? The host supposed the one who owed the most would love the creditor more. Jesus told him he answered correctly.

The difference between the man (i.e., the debtor owing the least) who hosted the dinner and the woman (i.e., the debtor owing the most) who attended the dinner is that the woman came to get her burden lifted. If you don't understand anything else about Jesus, do know that he is a burden-lifter and a heavy-load sharer. He will remove every hindering load and setback in your life. When the uninvited woman appeared at the dinner to which Jesus had been invited, she brought oil because she knew the oil applied in faith would break the burden of her debt. If you want a debilitating situation broken in your life, have oil at your table and don't be afraid to use it in faith to the glory of Jesus. The failures and setbacks in her life set her up for a comeback in life.

You prepare a table before me
in the presence of my enemies.
You anoint my head with oil;
my cup overflows.
—Psalm 23:5

Despite all that could be said about her, the often maligned woman in Luke's gospel quite possibly had incredible faith in scripture, for there is a Messianic prophecy that says the Messiah will give "[t]he oil of joy for mourning" (Isaiah 61:3). Oil, applied in faith—be it in your cooking or in your worship—aligns us with what is the Lord's, and the burden that is ours becomes His. In fact, the psalmist does say God gives us "oil" to make our faces shine, not in the sense of being oily, but in the sense of being the objects of His love and care (Psalm 104:15).

> OIL, APPLIED IN FAITH—BE IT IN YOUR COOKING OR IN YOUR WORSHIP—ALIGNS US WITH WHAT IS THE LORD'S, AND THE BURDEN THAT IS OURS BECOMES HIS.

As a pastor, I am often quite amused by the many different stories people share about their lives. Once a single mother shared with me that she used to anoint her sons' heads every morning before they left the house to go to the bus stop. One morning, when her dear sons had grown into teenagers, they resisted having her anoint their heads.

After about thirty minutes, she recounted, of chasing them around the house and wrestling with them to put some oil on their foreheads, she finally asked in exhaustion why they didn't want their heads anointed. It had been perfectly fine before she thought. The oldest spoke up and said, "Momma, we can pray for ourselves. Besides, we are tired of people teasing us every morning for having greasy heads."

Like a dutiful and faithful parent, God uses oil because good oil is good for us in so many ways. As a symbol of the Holy Spirit, oil is used to anoint us. Moreover, coupled with prayer, oil likewise becomes an agent of healing (James 5:14).

So, when you invite the Lord to your table, don't forget the oil. It's the right thing to have to get the breakthrough you want. God shouldn't have to chase you in order to bless you.

People close to me know that I am a popcorn lover; in all honesty, I fancy myself as a popcorn aficionado (whatever that is). But I'm old school, so I don't have much time for that modern, microwavable stuff. I like to get out my favorite old pot and pop it the natural way. It reminds me, I suppose, of my grandmother standing over her old Frigidaire® stove popping corn in the evening to get her five grandkids to quiet down so she wouldn't go crazy.

One evening after having finished everything, I decided to pop some popcorn as is my typical late-night habit. I put some oil in the old pot, measured in the right amount of corn, set the heat on medium, and went in another room to listen for it to start popping. After a while, I felt something was wrong. I could hear the corn popping, but something was awry. After a couple of minutes, I felt I'd better go check. I couldn't believe it. In my haste to get my popcorn started, I had forgotten to put the lid on the pot. What was missing was that I wasn't hearing the popped corn hit the lid. My popcorn had popped, but it was all over the stovetop and the floor. I never benefitted from the food.

Having the right oil is like having the lid on the pot. People don't think about the type of oil they use with their food, and although they may be attempting to eat healthily, if it is not being cooked in good oil, then the benefit of the food is lost. For instance, "Many people think canola oil is healthy due to savvy marketing, but it is not your best choice."[18] There

---

[18] Grace, Tabitha. "Oils: Everybody, clap your hands! Tasty, satiating fats are good for you." *The Power of Superfoods*. October 2017, p. 48.

are some much better choices. Quality oils, however, are vital to a healthy diet.

Many of us are like Simon, the man who invited Jesus to dinner; we forget the oil. There are some extremely good and healthy oils to have at the table and there are some not so good choices for oils; here are a few of the healthiest.

Oil	Benefits	Preparation
Olive Oil	• Fights heart disease • Fights cancer • Fights inflammation • Reduces risk of strokes • Lowers blood pressure • Fights weight gain • Fights Type 2 diabetes	• Cook • Natural
Sunflower Oil	• Promotes heart health • Lowers cholesterol • Beautifies skin • Boosts energy • Fights inflammation • Strengthens immune system • Fights cancer	• Cook • Natural

Oil	Benefits	Preparation
Avocado Oil	• Improves heart health • Improves eye health • Relieves osteoarthritis • Beautifies skin • Helps with weight loss • Detoxifies the body • Nourishes hair	• Cook • Natural
Coconut Oil	• Helps grow hair • Strengthens immune system • Speeds healing • Kills (certain) viruses • Lowers blood sugar • Promotes mental health	• Cook • Natural

SHE CALLED HIM "LORD"

A dear friend and colleague once asked me, "What would a meal look like if God prepared it?" I honestly didn't have an answer. The profundity of the question left me speechless. Indeed, what would a meal prepared by God look like? I long pondered the thought after his question.

All the same, the one thing I'm fairly certain of is that whatever the Lord prepares would be more than just food. It would constitute so much more, perhaps even the miraculous. Take, for instance, the mother who found Jesus, fell at his feet, and then begged him to cast the demon out of her daughter.

THE CHILDREN'S CRUMBS

Jesus left that place and went to the vicinity of Tyre. He entered a house and did not want anyone to know it; yet he could not keep his presence secret. In fact, as soon as she heard about him, a woman whose little daughter was possessed by an evil spirit came and fell at his feet. The woman was a Greek, born in Syrian Phoenicia. She begged Jesus to drive the demon out of her daughter.

"First let the children eat all they want," he told her, "for it is not right to take the children's bread and toss it to their dogs."

"Yes, Lord," she replied, "but even the dogs under the table eat the children's crumbs."

Then he told her, "For such a reply, you may go; the demon has left your daughter."

She went home and found her child lying on the bed, and the demon gone.

Mark 7:24–30 (NIV)

At first, Jesus rebuffed the mother; he explained that to take food away from the children for whom it was intended was not right, only to then have him humiliate her by referring to her and her demon-possessed daughter as "dogs." However, the woman's faith-laced retort, "Yes, Lord . . . but even the dogs under the table eat the children's crumbs," moved Jesus to speak healing into her life, and at the very moment he spoke it, her daughter was healed and set free.

What was it about the bread that the woman would so readily accept the children's crumbs, and exactly what did she say that moved Jesus to release healing power into the life of her child?

Interestingly, Jesus drew upon a metaphor to characterize her request as interrupting and besieging a meal intended for God's children, thus intimating that God uses food in ways other than simply eating to quell hunger.

The woman came seeking healing for her daughter, and Jesus in effect told her the healing is in the bread, but the bread is for my children, thus establishing the fact that God uses food to heal the people He loves. As pointed out in Chapter 3, for instance, God has often used bread (e.g., barley) to produce mighty miracles for the faithful. So, how do we access the Lord's miracle-working power in food?

Looking, again, at the story of the woman who desperately wanted her little girl freed from demon-possession, notice that she replied to Jesus, "Yes, Lord, . . . but even the dogs under the table eat the children's crumbs." A casual reading of the account suggests the woman's wit was what touched Jesus and moved him to heal her child. But frankly such an understanding scares me because that would suggest her quick-wittedness got her what she wanted from the Master.

It looks like that because she matched wits with the great teacher that she got her breakthrough. If that were the case, then many of us would go home from an encounter with Jesus just like we arrived. Personally, it usually takes me too long sometimes to come up with the perfect or witty answer in such situations, but there are some people I have known who have a sharp tongue. They can get you straight as it were before you even realize what hit you, and by the time you think of a comeback, the ordeal is over, and they are gone.

However, the Holy Spirit showed me that it was not her wit that touched and subsequently moved Jesus. On the contrary, what moved the carpenter's son from Nazareth was that she called him "Lord." The prophet Joel says, "And everyone who calls on the name of the Lord will be saved" (Joel 2:32). That woman knew enough about God's word to call Jesus "Lord," and when she did, what started out as willingness to accept crumbs became a buffet of blessings in her life and in the life of her daughter.

Invoke "the name of the Lord" over your bread, and you can expect the miraculous benefits of bread to be released in your life.

> INVOKE "THE NAME OF THE LORD" OVER YOUR BREAD, AND YOU CAN EXPECT THE MIRACULOUS BENEFITS OF BREAD TO BE RELEASED IN YOUR LIFE.

Whole Grain	Benefits	Preparation
Barley	• Maintains a healthy colon • Fights toxins • Ensures strong bones • Promotes youthful appearance of skin • Helps control cholesterol • Lowers blood sugar • Prevents cancer	• Boil • Bake

LOOK BETTER. FEEL BETTER. LIVE BETTER.

Whole Grain	Benefits	Preparation
Wheat*	• Prevents Type 2 diabetes • Reduces blood estrogen • Fights breast cancer • Fights heart disease • Reduces inflammation	• Bake • Boil
Sorghum	• Reduces risk of cancer • Controls diabetes • Boosts energy • Prevents arthritis • Fights anemia	• Toasted • Popped • Baked
Oats	• Lowers cholesterol • Lowers blood sugar • Beautifies skin • Lowers blood pressure • Strengthens immune system	• Topical treatment • Baking • Smoothies
Maize (Corn)	• Fights tumors • Fights heart disease • Lowers cholesterol • Lowers blood pressure • Promotes healthy skin • Strengthens immune system • Lowers blood sugar	• Steam • Bake • Grill

Whole Grain	Benefits	Preparation
Rice	• Lowers blood pressure • Prevents cancer (i.e., brown rice) • Promotes healthy skin • Lowers cholesterol • Fights heart disease	• Steam • Topical treatment • Rice water

* *Always check with a physician before consuming large amounts of wheat.*

If the children's crumbs from that meal would heal a demon-possessed child, then the children for whom the meal is intended should expect even more in the way of miraculous benefits and healing power. When she called him "Lord," the woman was saying, "Jesus, I'm your child, too, and I'm entitled to a blessing and a breakthrough, too." At that very hour, her request was granted. When God gets ready to bless you, He can do it in a hurry. You are entitled to a miracle. Claim it!

A crumb from the Lord has more healing and deliverance power than a banquet at the enemy's table. Eating God's way has benefits for the faithful to do exceedingly beyond what can be thought or imagined. Food experts are clear "if you incorporate more natural choices into your diet, you'll feel better, look better, and *be* [sic] better."[19]

> WHEN GOD GETS READY TO BLESS YOU, HE CAN DO IT IN A HURRY. YOU ARE ENTITLED TO A MIRACLE. CLAIM IT!"

---

[19] Friedlander, Steven, Editor-in-Chief. "You Are What You Eat: Part 1." *100 Ways to Live to 100: Expert Advice for a Longer Life.* July 2017, p. 72.

CLOSING PRAYER

My Lord and my God, I come to You as a stranger from a foreign land. Faith in You brought me out of darkness, and I come desiring healing and cleansing of my mind, body, and soul. Give me the faith to unlock the miracle-working power found in the food from Your table. As Your child, I claim right now the blessings and miracles in store for me and my life.

Amen.

Insights for Looking Better: _____

_____
_____
_____
_____
_____
_____
_____
_____
_____
_____
_____

THE CHILDREN'S CRUMBS

Insights for Feeling Better: _____

LOOK BETTER. FEEL BETTER. LIVE BETTER.

Insights for Living Better:

Epilogue

SLAY IT

Sin is a destroyer. It will tear up everything it comes in contact with, and it will ravage every place it is allowed to linger, so getting sin out of your life, in any form, is not just necessary for health and wellness, it is absolutely critical.

Most of us, however, have been so duped by sin and its consequences that we naively incubate in our lives what's meant to destroy us when we should be slaying it. Like a beautiful and innocent finch will hatch the egg of a murderous cowbird, we safely harbor harmful things in our lives that if left unchecked will push out the healthy and good things God has for us. Sin won't wear suspicious clothes and won't drive a big black car with tinted windows. It will often appear as innocuous as an egg in a nest, and while we're looking for the bad guy, destruction is as close to us and as guarded as the food on our plates.

This book is not a diet book or a cook book so much as it is an eye-opener meant to bring awareness to the benefits of whole and godly foods and to signal alarm to harmful dietary habits that are doing tremendous harm to our bodies and to our health.

God sent me this revelation to tell you that He wants to heal you. He is your Healer, and if you will put your trust in Him with the food you eat, He will show you how much He loves you and wants you to look, feel, and live better according to His plan for your life. The Lord is your Healer, so slay it.

SCRIPTURE MEDITATIONS

1 Corinthians 10:31	84
Daniel 1:18–20	80
Isaiah 1:19	74
Isaiah 55:2	9
Jeremiah 31:14	61
Joel 2:19	67
Matthew 6:31–33	26
Proverbs 13:25	24
Psalm 23:5	92
Psalm 107:9	45
Psalm 145:15–16	49

ADDITIONAL RESOURCES

Buettner, Dan. *The Blue Zones Solution: Eating and Living Like the World's Healthiest People.* National Geographic Partners, LLC, 2015.

Greger, Michael, with Gene Stone. *The How Not To Die Cookbook: 100+ Recipes to Help Prevent and Reverse Disease.* First Edition. Flatiron Books, 2017.

Morris, Martha Clare. *Diet For The Mind: The Latest Science on What to Eat to Prevent Alzheimer's and Cognitive Decline—from the Creator of the Mind Diet.* First Edition. Little, Brown and Company, 2017.

Oz, Dr. Mehmet C. *Food Can Fix It: The Superfood Switch to Fight Fat, Defy Aging, and Eat Your Way Healthy.* 1st ed. Simon & Schuster, Inc., 2017.

Segal, Eran, Eran Elinav, with Eve Adamson. *The Personalized Diet: The Pioneering Program to Lose Weight and Prevent Disease.* First Edition. Grand Central Publishing, 2017.

Smith, Laura Harris. *The Healthy Living Handbook: Simple, Everyday Habits for Your Body, Mind and Spirit.* Chosen Books, 2017.

Warren, Rick, Daniel Amen, Mark Hyman, with Sean Foy and Dee Eastman. *The Daniel Plan: 40 Days to a Healthier Life.* Zondervan, 2013.

ABOUT THE AUTHOR

As an award-winning seminarian of the Divinity School at Duke University, Derrick Justice was once asked to write an article for publication in the school newsletter; ultimately, he penned an insightful essay on the idiosyncrasies and similarities between good cooking and effective preaching, earning him rave reviews from his peers and many of his professors.

Earlier in his academic career at Virginia Commonwealth University in Richmond, Virginia, Dr. Justice was partly able to put himself through college advising friends and classmates on how to eat and take vitamins properly to successfully rid themselves of acne and other unwanted skin blemishes. To those he helped, he just had a gift for understanding the relationship between food and healing.

Years later, as the single parent of two sons, Joshua and Joseph, Derrick A. Justice's skills in the kitchen allowed him to raise two healthy and sound young men on nutritious food, coupled with creative life themes—and quite a few tall tales, that today is the source of much family amusement as they fondly look back on those trying times.

Unbeknownst to him, the Lord was molding and shaping his life and ministry to one day articulate the life-changing benefits of faith and food—evident in his doctoral dissertation: Family Meal Plan: A Post Modern Approach to Healing the Disrupted Family.

Today, as the Senior Pastor of Lillington Star F.W.B. Church in the beautiful city of Lillington, North Carolina, D.A. Justice's messages and workshops on faith, food, and healing are revelatory, changing lives and altering eating behaviors to promote the quality of life God's people long for and deeply desire.